Nine Friends

Jeannie

Nine Friends

in time of loss

Jeannie Seeley-Smith

gfp

NINE FRIENDS IN TIME OF LOSS
SECOND EDITION

Published by Garden Fleetfoot Press
PO Box 6, Gulliver, Michigan 49508
www.gardenfleetfoot.com

Cover design by Jim Villaflores
Interior design by Gram Telen

Publisher Data:
Seeley-Smith, Jeannie
Nine Friends – In Time of Loss / By Jeannie Seeley-Smith. –
Gulliver : Garden Fleetfoot Press. 2017
62 p: 18.5 cm.
ISBN-10: 0-9762544-3-3
ISBN-13: 978-0-9762544-3-0
1 . Loss (Psychology)
2 . Metaphor (Literature)

Printed in the United States of America
10 9 8 7 6 5 4 3 2 1

In memory of my mother, whom I lost at age nine.
She was forty-one.
And to my children and grandchildren whom
she would have dearly loved.

Acknowledgments

I am deeply thankful for the love, encouragement, and wisdom of my husband and best friend, Gary, who during the initial drafts would give thumbs up or thumbs down. Right from the beginning, I trusted his insight, editing, and literary knowledge. Philosophically, I have always been his student. Therefore, this book would never have been written without his continual belief that I was writing something of value.

I owe tremendous gratitude to my creative editor and brother, Gary Shoup, author of *Suma the Elephant*. His skillful editing so beautifully blends with my own voice that I can no longer distinguish his words from mine. From the beginning to the end, he encouraged me to trust in myself, to believe in my work, and to recognize that I held some magic, at least he thought I did, which eventually helped me to believe it myself.

I thank my darling, lifelong friend, Sue Zelickson, one of the first readers to encourage me, giving me the motivation to continue writing. She continues to be my inspiration to this day. I am grateful to my two fabulous sister-in-law's, Kathleen Shoup, who read early drafts after she lost her beloved mother, and encouraged me over and over to have the work published. And Newt Shoup, who continues to teach me about gratefulness, contentment, and sacrificial love.

I am so thankful to my twin sister and soulmate, Kathy, who for years would relentlessly ask, "When are you going to write another book? When are you going to write another book?" Okay, I heard you.

Postscript: Two years and one day after *Nine Friends* was first published I lost my twin, Kathy. It was a fourteen month battle during which time I never gave up hope that together we would triumph over her cancer. But, in the end, it was not meant to be. Without the help of my nine friends, I don't know if I would have made it.

Preface

It's nearly impossible to find a human being who does not experience the fear of losing someone or something they love. Some have terrible anxiety over this looming destiny, while others don't fuss much about it at all, but eventually, we all ask ourselves, "Will I survive?" Simply put, Loss is as much a part of existence as life itself. In the flash of a moment, everything that's important to us could be gone. We are grateful if Loss does not come suddenly, but even if not, one day, family, friends, jobs, homes, pets, possessions, and a host of other situations will come to an end. We either say good-bye or they do. It's the downside of life.

Now, here's the good news! In times of Loss, there are nine friends who emerge. If only we knew their value from the get-go, we would not resist them to the extent that we do, for they are truly lifesavers. In this little book, we will meet them. Even though four of them are particularly unpleasant, each one is essential to our process.

In the end, we'll all look back and be amazed at how well our nine friends worked together to help us through. Who would have thought that because of these friends, we are capable of rising from the ashes of our loss like the legendary phoenix: wiser, more compassionate, more peaceful, and with a deeper level of consciousness?

As we come to know these friends, we'll be fascinated by their timing, for it appears that each one knows exactly when they are needed—and *exactly* the right time to hand us off to the next one.

How do they know how to do this? It's hard to deny that it all appears to be part of a greater plan—a plan, if not derailed by our Foes, can lead us into a life-changing transformation.

Shock

Summer: Nighttime
House lights on thunderstorm rages,
lightning bolt hits house

From out of the blue comes a shattering bolt! A devastating Loss hits. "Oh my God! Oh, no! How can this be happening?! Oh, please, *please*, God! No!" Our internal switchboard immediately dials 911. "Help—Help! Does anyone hear me? Oh, please, someone help me! *Please* tell me it's not true!" In horror, we shout to the heavens, "What have *you* done?"

We stagger, intoxicated with disbelief. Looking up, we yell, "Where are those awful sounds coming from?" Terror grips us as we realize they are coming from us. Piercing cries, so earsplitting we barely hear the knock at the door. Frozen from fright, unable to move, the knock gives way to pounding. As our knees weaken, we grab the edge of the wall. Just as we are about to collapse, the door flies open. Our first friend enters. Dressed in a baggy combat medic uniform, *Shock* arrives bent over and panting from his forced break-in. Through blurred vision, we notice he has two hefty knapsacks slung over his small back: one red, one yellow.

"Get out!" we scream.

Unimpressed by our protest, *Shock* gets right to work. He drops to his knees and dumps out all the contents from the red knapsack. Our eyes grow wide as we stare at terrifying vials rolling around like colorful marbles at our feet. *Shock*, knowing time is of an essence, grabs one of the vials and straightaway administers a numbing potion, a cognitive anesthesia. It works fast. Our thought process is gone. *Shock's* second potion numbs our muscles. Our movements are halted to *snail's pace*.

Now digging deep into the yellow knapsack, *Shock* comes up with a third potion. This one spins us into "nowhere zone." Our nerves are deadened. We no longer feel. Our eyes glaze over; mercifully our mind and body shuts down. *Shock*, finally satisfied with the success of his initial maneuvers, begins to secure our house. Paralyzed, unable to comprehend, we stand and watch *Shock* rush around tacking up "Out of Order" signs. "What is he doing?" we agonize.

Unbeknownst to us, the posted signs are intended to keep our Foes at bay—scary, toothy, snarling Foes who are beginning to circle. One such Foe, sadistic *Fear,* has already found a crack and, like a wily snake, slithers through.

"Gotcha!" he hisses!

Fear's purpose is to destroy us. His sleazy desire is to rip away our sanity, conceivably our life. If allowed to take over during our collapsed state, *Fear* can panic us into destructive behavior or, worse yet, permanently rob us of our minds. *Fear* has even been known to stop beating hearts.

Shock works at record speed to stop this internal attack. By first shutting us down, he is buying time until we're ready to absorb the horrendous reality of our Loss. His posted signs, in our paralyzed state, cleverly creates the appearance that no one's home. As we stumble around in a trance, *Fear* becomes disillusioned. Unfortunately for him, we're too numb to feel his presence. "Darn!" he snarls. Because of *Shock*'s ingenious strategies, *Fear* is unable to fulfill his nefarious plans. For the time—thwarted, he slithers back out to find other quarry. He'll be back.

At the end of round 1, we're surprised to discover we're still breathing, if only barely. What we don't realize quite yet is that we can thank our good friend *Shock* that we've made it through this far. *Shock* kept us from absorbing the full impact of our horrific Loss. He knows that there are plenty of days ahead for us to process, but not just now. We need time.

Shock's tremendous power is exhausting and difficult to maintain. For that reason, he doesn't hang around for long—maybe a couple of days, perhaps a bit longer—but while he's with us, he has complete control, never leaving us for a moment. He wraps a cloak of protection around us so tightly; we lose sight of the sunrises and sunsets. The numbing potions are so intense that we are no longer conscious of voices and movements surrounding us, including our own. Nonetheless, it is all part of *Shock*'s plan. Despite the fact that we loathe him, he still protects us from harm in his own strange but efficient way.

Oh no! The unspeakable has returned! *Shock*'s potions are starting to wear off and the terrible truth is sinking in. *Fear* is back, and our excruciating Loss is crashing in around us, once again. Fortunately, our good friend *Shock* is well aware of the situation; in fact, he's been expecting it. Indeed, he's been preparing for it! The return of our awful reality signals that his time is coming to an end, and he begins to pack up. He must leave so that another friend can take his place. In fact, she's headed up the path, right now.

Hastily, *Shock* gathers up his "Out of Order" signs, folds up his protective cloak, tightens the caps to his potions, and stuffs it all back in his knapsacks. Now, with one great heave, he swings the huge load onto his tiny back and he's out the door. However, he won't go far. He'll stand outside on the porch for a while, just in case he needs to jump back in, but he won't get comfortable. He has no intention of hanging around. For the most part, his purpose is done. And after a few days, he will be heading down the path never to return again.

Oh, if only it were so.

On his way out, his head bumps into the knees of our second friend, who is already on our porch—a friend we will come to despise.

Sob

Summer: Nighttime
House lights on but very dim
Storming, trees' limbs are bent over from the heavy rain

Contrary to *Shock*, *Sob* has no intention of knocking. She penetrates through the door like a ghostly vapor. As the haunting mist begins to take shape, an image forms that is petrifying, but strangely, it's also reassuring. Draped in a loin cloth and carrying a suspiciously overflowing knapsack, *Sob* is gigantic, towering over us by several feet. As we look up at her, our initial tinge of reassurance vanishes and we begin to shake.

It takes us seconds to realize that *Shock* and *Sob* could not be more different. And it's not only about size. Whereas *Shock* enveloped us in his protective cloak, shutting down our feelings, *Sob* works like a crowbar and pries them wide open, exposing gaping wounds. We must be aware that these wounds are not just the old run-of-the-mill cuts and bruises! Oh no, these wounds caused by the poisonous arrows of unacceptable Loss and unparalleled heartbreak are bleeding profusely. There are no other human wounds that come close to their severity.

Sob knows that the unmerciful bleeding of our tears is the only way to rid us of the insufferable poisons. Therefore, during this time, she leaves the arrows in place, causing us uncontrollable weeping. In her compassion, however, she provides the venom with a second escape route. *Sob* gives us a voice that shatters mirrors. As our howls increase in volume, the venom erupts and the deep purging begins. It's not a pretty sight, nor is it meant to be.

As from a distance, we hear a dreadful moaning arise deep within us—a place we never knew existed. This tortured sound is accompanied by other frightful changes within our body. Our breathing is constricted, our throat is frozen, and it's impossible to speak. We wail with a noise so guttural, so foreign, we feel separate from it. It's as if we are standing outside staring at ourselves in astonishment—so far removed, we fear we'll never return.

Coming in convulsive waves, crashing ashore like a monstrous storm, *Sob* batters us until we curl up into a helpless ball. When her hammering finally diminishes, we are left physically ill and mentally exhausted. Then *Sob*, similar to *Shock*, administers a soothing potion, and for a short period, we escape into a shallow sleep. When we awake, we think it's all been a dream. Then boom! The chilling reality sets in again as lurking *Fear* finds another crack. Once again, *Sob* takes control. *Fear,* no match for *Sob,* slinks away.

Going through this hellish ordeal, we can scarcely believe that *Sob* is our friend, but she is. *Sob* is so eager to rid our body of pain that she may push us farther than what we're capable of enduring—or so it seems. But we must learn to trust her. Keeping our wounds open and the arrows in place (for a time) is essential to our healing, and the sooner we stop fighting *Sob*, the faster the toxic venom will escape. But oh, the agony!

We now regret *Shock*'s departure. At least when *he* was with us, we felt separated from our dreadful reality. *Shock* also came and left quickly. *Sob*, on the other hand, appears to have no intention of letting up or leaving. However, there is one positive change. During this time, *Sob* had shrunk to normal size. She no longer towers over us. Now fitting comfortably in our overstuffed chair, she seems to have settled in—for what? Forever?

Finally, after several days of misery, *Sob* starts extracting the arrows and the bleeding lessens. Sympathetically, *Sob* steps back and gives us a reprieve. She knows we need rest. Caution: we must not to be fooled. There is more to come. But for now, *Sob* yields and takes up residence out on the porch swing.

Time passes. Long days fade into even longer nights of restless sleep. As we toss and turn, we can hear her rocking back and forth—humming and waiting. Over the hinges, eerie squeaking sounds, *Sob* calls out, "Don't worry! I'm here, and I'm not going anywhere! You still need me!"

The battle begins. We simply don't want *Sob* lurking around anymore. Yes, we're grateful she has removed some of the arrows, but enough is enough, we want to be done with her. "Go away!" we scream. *Sob*, patiently swinging, is unmoved. She pushes herself back with one foot and then with the other, all while gazing at the sky. "Why won't she stop that maddening humming?" we silently moan. *Sob* just waits. She knows it won't be long before she needs to reenter. We know she's wrong. We don't *need* anyone, least of all *her*!

Oh, if only it were so.

Long weeks turn into a month, and then we hear a tapping at the door. *Sob's* patience is gone. She wants back in. Just thinking about her gut-wrenching tactics makes us shake. If we let her back in, we are sure the bleeding will start up again, and she'll never leave. So we run over and latch the door. No luck! She has the key. We lean our back against the door and push. She pushes back. We dig in our heels. Again, no luck! Our shoes leave skid marks on the wood floor as she pushes the door wide open. She has us in her grasp. We surrender.

Our face drops down into our hands. We collapse to our knees. Our thoughts flee as our body wracks with an explosion of tears. Once again, our cries mimic waves crashing ashore. We're in a typhoon. Our eyes and nose are fountains. Venomous fluids flow out of us as our voice pierces the air in agony. The all too familiar wailing begins again, and we gasp for breath. Oh, how we loathe *Sob*!

Exhausted, we collapse into sleep—restless sleep, on and off for days. Then one morning, we awake and are surprised to notice a slight feeling of freshness. Something different has happened—a shift, not much, just a bit. During our sleep, *Sob* must have wrenched more arrows from our wounds. We're inching forward. It's lifting. Oh, there is no doubt that the wounds are still wide open, but a few scabs are forming.

It is here that we begin to realize that our emotionally pain-inflicting *Sob* is helping us through our torment. So we make a deal with her. We promise not to hate her anymore. She can hang out on the porch swing as long as she wants. We even tell her that from now on, whenever she knocks, we will let her back in without a struggle. In turn, *Sob* promises to only come in when we most need her. True, we'll never be glad to see her, but we are no longer frightened of her because, well, *Sob* is actually a good friend after all. In retrospect, she's proved herself to be very effective, compassionate, and much wiser than we first thought. And although we don't realize it at the time, *Sob* has prepared us for our next two friends.

Unfortunately, we won't like them any more than the first two.

Grief and Sorrow

Autumn: Nighttime
Lights are out with the exception of one lone porch light
Trees still hold on to a few dead leaves—
most have fallen to the ground

Ding dong, ding dong! The tolling of distant bells announces the arrival of our next two visitors. Appearing as shrouded monks, they trudge slowly up the beaten path toward our home. *Shock* is gone. *Sob* is still here, but the squeak is gone. She now quietly rocks back and forth on the porch swing as our next two friends climb the front steps. How rude! They pass through the door without even a cursory knock.

Lying feebly on the couch, we're so exhausted we can't even lift ourselves up enough to protest. Their faces are grim and pale, giving them a dolorous, ill-humored appearance.

They introduce themselves: two brothers—twins—named *Grief* and *Sorrow*.

"Oh, great—twins," we groan. We sense double trouble. Through swollen, puffed-up eyes, we notice that they are exactly the same size. They are tall, slim built with full beards, dressed in long black velvet cloaks. They peer at us over their round, green spectacles perched on the tips of their noses. Claiming they are practitioners, *Grief* taps on his knapsack and explains he cares for the body. *Sorrow* says his knapsack is filled with paraphernalia that works on our emotions.

"Huh? What? Who sent for you? Go away!" we snarl. "I don't need either of you!"

Oh, if only it were so.

Hoarse from the pummeling of *Sob*, incapable of further protesting, we watch silently as they start to rearrange our house for what's to come. As if preparing for a horrendous storm, they move from room to room, shutting doors, slamming down windows, and latching up shutters. We moan as the soothing breezes that were once flowing through our cozy house are gone. They show no pity as they now tack up heavy black curtains to block out the sun. After closing up the house, they hide our books, turn off the music, flip off the lights, throw out the firewood, and take away our food. We are convinced they are sadists. Everything that could make life tolerable is gone. Our inner light flickers out and we're engulfed in darkness.

As *Grief* and *Sorrow* settle in, taking up residence in our mind, body, and spirit, we abandon the couch to take refuge in bed, moaning deeply as we crawl under the blankets. Oh my, *Grief* and *Sorrow* are heavy! When we were so encompassed by *Sob*, we were barely conscious of our heartbeat, but now, every beat is painful. The Twins are merciless as they stab at our broken heart with pitchforks—constantly, day and night. There is no relief.

Because their assaults exact a major toll on our body, we have no strength to fight back. We groan as we roll over and over in our bed, trying to find a cool, soft place that would provide the tiniest bit of relief, but there is none. We think we might die. At times, we wish we could.

Eventually, we pull ourselves out of bed, and in doing so, we pass a mirror. We see a face we don't recognize. We step back and stare. "Who is that strained, saggy-cheeked, worn-out person?" we ask. Dull, empty eyes stare back at us beneath droopy lids and unkempt hair. "I am you," the reflection answers. Our smile, considered one of our best features, is now a lifeless frozen line drawn on a face without spirit. We retreat back to our bed and, once again, pull the blankets up over our head.

Life takes on an unfamiliar tempo. We struggle through the days, doing nothing more than our body demands. *Grief* and *Sorrow* are our constant companions. "When will you go?" we ask them. There's no answer. Our flesh and blood friends stop by now and then, but soon find out that we're no longer any fun. We have nothing to give them and nothing pleasant to say. "Just go away," we silently plead. They read our expression, quickly make their apologies, and leave. We can't blame them. Who would want to keep company with us and the Terrible Twins?

How is it, anyway, we complain, that the Twins dare call themselves *friends*? Aren't friends supposed to make you feel better? "You feel like Foes!" we yell at them. "Your pain is unbearable. For god's sake! When will you leave?" Again—no answer.

We are not aware of it, but *Grief* and *Sorrow* are *not* the ones wielding the pitchforks. The excruciating pain is coming from the barbs of Loss's heartbreaking arrows that continue to pierce at us. Regrettably, depending on the extent of our Loss, it can take a considerable time to stop the hemorrhaging.

What we don't know, as yet, is that *Grief* and *Sorrow* are, in fact, healers. For sure, they are mournful creatures, but they are definitely our friends. Their work is essential to our eventual healing, and without them, we can't move forward. Yes, *Grief* and *Sorrow* are masterminds. And their tactics are essential to the healing process. And like all good friends, they will stay with us for as long as we need them, even though we tell them over and over again, "Just go!"

Weeks may turn into months and, depending on the depth of our Loss, months can turn into a year or more. Then one day, a stream of sunlight breaks through a crack in the shutter. We do a double-take to confirm. Yes, it's definitely sunlight! We manage a tiny smile. Soon after, we become conscious of hunger pains. We take a deep breath. We know we're still some distance from being healed, but an appetite is encouraging. We also notice that our heartbeats are not as excruciating. Furthermore, we have come to realize how much we need *Grief* and *Sorrow.* We recognize that they brought us through, and that because of them, we are on the other side. There is hope. So now we ask ourselves whether we need our twins anymore. Perhaps, they too have realized it's time to move on. But uh-oh—there's a problem.

Every so often, *Grief* and *Sorrow* can get so wrapped up in their healing process that they forget it's time to leave. Yes, if we're not careful, they can become *too* comfortable. To make matters worse, so can we. Eventually, we might even resign ourselves to believing that we're the Three Musketeers! That's not good, and if this precarious situation occurs, we need to act quickly to rectify it.

We must be careful not to get to a place where we wallow around with *Grief* and *Sorrow* just for the fellowship. Overstaying their usefulness not only delays our other friends' arrival, it creates an environment that attracts Foes—not only *Fear*, but other life-sucking Foes like *Guilt* and *Self-Pity*—all of them *very* dangerous! Left to their own devices, they will drag us down into a deep, dark tunnel, stealing all the progress we've made thus far. So if a year or more has passed and we're still hanging out with *Grief* and *Sorrow*, it's probably time to plan their farewell party.

We start by looking in the mirror. What do we see? Yes, we see great sadness, but we no longer see the look of devastation staring back at us. We're stronger now. Our will is back. We've regained confidence. We take a moment to relish these changes, then we open the front door and step out onto the porch. We call to the twins to join us. Once they're out of the house, we say, "Thank you," and hug them good-bye. After a tearful farewell, we go back inside and close the door behind us. We take a deep breath. It feels good. We know that we're free to move on. However, we are under no illusion that *Grief* and *Sorrow* are gone forever. For some of us, *Grief* and *Sorrow* may always share our porch swing with *Sob*. But for now, they are out of sight, out of mind, and a tremendous weight is lifted. Maybe it's over. Maybe, this is it. It certainly feels like a new beginning. But we know deep inside—it's not over. There's more.

Our next friend has been patiently camping out beside the path for some time. He begins to stir and slowly starts to break camp. After leisurely rolling up his bedroll, he takes down his tent and gathers up his supplies. His knapsack packed, he meanders up the path toward our house.

It's been a long wait. *Acceptance* finally arrives.

Acceptance

Winter: Daylight
Cloudy but peeks of sun
Heavy white snow on house, ground and trees,
house path is shoveled

The frustrating situation with *Acceptance* is that he's old and pokey, and when he eventually does show up, we're exhausted. But to his credit, when he enters our house, we immediately sense a renewed strength. Nevertheless, we still can only manage a meager welcome.

Acceptance doesn't appear to mind our lack of exuberance, as he too only gives us an acknowledging nod as he saunters in dragging his heavy knapsack. We are greatly relieved to see that he is dressed comfortably in casual jeans, a heavy wool vest, colorful scarf, plaid shirt, and hiking boots. We notice his ample white hair falls out of his fur ear-flap hat.

We begin thinking this friend could actually be tolerable. However, still drained, it takes us some time to prepare his room. We shuffle around slowly, hindered by the fact that we don't know the first thing about *Acceptance* and have no clue as to what he likes. It would help, of course, if *Acceptance* pitched in, but he is a bit of a slacker and seems to expect us to do all the work. That's okay. We feel so much more productive now that *Grief* and *Sorrow* are out of the house.

Our effort, scanty as it is, soon pays off. After just a few days, we notice that *Acceptance*'s presence has given us new vigor. Each day, we're gaining strength. And now we actually find enjoyment in caring for him. We even bake cookies—the first batch since our Loss. The worst is over. From this point on, it's all uphill!

Oh, if only it were so.

About the time *Acceptance* completely unpacks and settles in, something happens. It's not a "good" something, and in fact, it jeopardizes the entire purpose of *Acceptance's* arrival. It appears that *Acceptance* is much more powerful than he had initially let on. And unfortunately, this power is a challenge to one of our most ancient and truculent Foes—evil *Anger*—the nemesis of *Acceptance*. Ever since *Acceptance* has settled in, *Anger* has been circling the house, swishing her scaly tail and salivating at the thought of throwing him out. Oh yes, she's planning a coup d'état. It's why she's come. It's what she lives for.

She now begins to make her move. In her typical sneaky fashion, *Anger* creeps in through the back door and heads right for *Acceptance's* room. She finds it empty and slips inside. Once in, she turns the deadbolt. "Hee-hee-hee," she smirks. The first stage of the infiltration is accomplished. The second stage is letting us know she plans to stay.

"How dare *Anger* try to evict *Acceptance*!" we stamp around shouting. "Just who does she think she is, anyway?" But then we think again. "Wait a doggone moment! What's the matter with *Acceptance*? Why isn't *he* pounding on the door? Why is *he* not standing next to me, putting up a fight to get his room back?" At this point, conceding that *Acceptance* is probably hiding behind the couch, we determine to go it alone. So with as much strength as we're able to muster, we fling open the door to confront *Anger*.

Amused, *Anger* creeps right up next to us and whispers in our ear, "Stick with me. I'm your *real* friend. I'll make you stronger and give you more control over your life than your weak-kneed, namby-pamby *Acceptance* friend ever dreamed of. Let's kick him out. He doesn't belong." *Anger* talks fast. She knows she has only a small window of opportunity before *Acceptance's* presence shrouds us in serenity.

For a moment, we are tempted. We tell ourselves, "I certainly am entitled to rant and rave after what I have been through. In fact, I deserve as much of *Anger's* friendship as I can get! Besides, I love the power and control *Anger* gives me. *Hmmm*, yes, indeed! I think I just might move *Anger* in!"

Danger! *Danger*! As tempted as we are, as much as we thirst for feelings of empowerment and control, as much as we feel we deserve to be rageful, we must fight back with all our strength. There is no doubt that *Ang*er intends to lead us into despair. We cannot give in!

So we have second thoughts. Fortunately, we're beginning to recognize Friends from Foes. We also eventually realize that it is not in *Acceptance's* nature to fight, and frankly, it's not his place to do so. Apparently, the job belongs to us to create an environment for *Acceptance* to stay. There is another good reason to give full support to *Acceptance*. *Anger* is a liar and a thief—an awful combination. Contrary to her shameless sweet talk, *Anger* does not, as promised, make us feel stronger or more powerful. In fact, she zaps our strength by tying up our emotions into one colossal, twisted knot, leaving us with our blood boiling, teeth and hands clenched, and head pounding. This despicable Foe also does not give us control. She steals it! Her wicked plan is to put us under *her* control, which then opens the door for other Foes, like *Bitterness* and *Hate*. After *Anger* provides our Foes with the red carpet treatment and declares her coup victorious, she intends to nail up the doors and bar the windows. She's got us!

Her ingenious strategy is all designed to keep out our other friends, still yet to come. With *Anger's* mission accomplished—well, welcome to the dark side. And down the road, if we ever do regain the strength to escape *Anger*, she will have left a trail of ruin so devastating, it will take a lifetime to recover. So we must resist, resist, *resist* evil *Anger*!

In the end, we decide against the darkness. Capitalizing on our renewed strength from *Acceptance*, we dig in and subdue our slippery Foe, *Anger*. We win the battle—at least for now. Humiliated, dragging her scaly tail behind her, *Anger* leaves. *Acceptance* is now serenely ensconced back in his room, munching on warm cookies.

Even though we know it was up to us to create this environment for *Acceptance*, we can't help but think that the whole battle scene would have been a heck of a lot easier if *Acceptance* had been a bit more assertive. However, what can we expect? By now, we already know we can't depend on *Acceptance* to jump in when the going gets rough. We remember how he took his good old sweet time showing up. We also recall how after moving in, he just kicked back while we ran around baking, fussing, and fluffing his pillows. And now, once again, we were the ones left alone brawling with *Anger?* Yes, we sort of realized it was our job. But why didn't he lend a hand? What's going on?

Ah-ha! It dawns on us.

Acceptance knew all along that he was fully capable of throwing *Anger* out, but he chose not to in order to help us realize that—even in our weakened state—we have choices. We think back on how *Shock*, *Sob*, and the terrible twins

Grief and *Sorrow* barged right in uninvited. We had no choice but to let them in. However, that was not the case with *Acceptance*. When *Acceptance* first arrived, we greeted him. Granted, not enthusiastically, but still, he has been the only friend so far that we prepared a room for. We also chose, over time, to make *Acceptance* feel welcome, and ultimately, it was our choice to reject *Anger*. The knowledge that we are making good choices during this confusing time rejuvenates our spirit and boosts our confidence that we can eventually survive our Loss. Yes, thanks to our good friend—kind, gentle, patient, lay-in-the-weeds *Acceptance*—we feel stronger and slightly more in control.

Acceptance, now fully aware that we've made our choice, begins to shake off his lethargic mood and starts to help out. He begins by unlatching the shutters, then he tears down the black curtains, and finally opens the windows! We breathe deeply, inhaling the scent of fresh air. We feel so grateful. Now our appetite returns, which helps us to regain strength. Next, he creates sounder sleep. Our thoughts become clearer. "What is this we're feeling?" we ask. Ah—yes, it's a sense of well-being. We had forgotten what it felt like.

Not long after, we wake up to freshly fallen snow. We dig out our heaviest coat, find our boots, grab our gloves, wrap a long scarf around our neck, and walk out the door. "Good morning!" we call out to *Sob*. "I won't be needing you today." We wade through the beautiful powder snow along the path in contentment, nonchalantly picking branches off the holly bushes for the kitchen windowsill. It's good to be alive.

Time passes by in leisurely fashion. Our days drift in and out. We continue to feel stronger. There is other good news. We are aware that we're thinking of things other than our Loss. We find that we're even making plans. We have been so self-absorbed for so long, it's time to think of others. We also notice something else: *Acceptance* is acting fidgety. We walk into his room one morning to find his knapsack half-packed. Is he leaving? Is this it?

One morning, as spring is arriving, we look out the window, and there's *Acceptance* with his knapsack fully packed, standing on the front porch gazing in the distance. In his characteristic fashion (after dropping his knapsack on a rocking chair), he walks slowly down the stairs, then ambles down the long path to greet someone.

A new friend has just rounded the bend, and *Acceptance* is heading out to meet her. We watch from a distance as they greet each other with a huge hug, and now together, they start back toward the house. We're intrigued because, as they approach, *Acceptance* begins to linger behind, but his companion quickens her pace. We feel *real* excitement for the first time since our Loss. Something wonderful is happening. As she gets closer, we notice she is carrying a large bundle that looks like a quilt. A small stack of fireplace wood protrudes from her knapsack. Balanced on her head is what looks like a hat. No, it's a teapot! A lovely English teapot!

Here comes *Comfort*!

Comfort

Spring: Sunrise
A beautiful morning glow
Trees, tulips, and lilacs are blooming

Oh, glory be! We fly off the porch running (after bumping into the porch swing and rocking chairs where *Sob, Grief,* and *Sorrow* are dozing) to hail our old friend!

"Hello, *Comfort*!" we yell. "Oh, I'm so happy to see you! You have finally returned!" Our eyes fill with tears. Exuberantly, attempting to avoid the firewood on her back, we wrap our arms around her. Her long white hair and round pudgy body is such a welcome sight, we simply cannot contain our enthusiasm! Her chubby rosy cheeks beam with a smile, warming us from head to toe. Her eyes sparkle as she greets us, "I am so pleased to be here! It has been a long time."

"Here, let me take the logs!" we exclaim. "I can also carry the quilt. I have been waiting for you for so long! Welcome home!" We continue to gush as we grab her knapsack and take the huge fluffy quilt from her hand.

"Oh, it's so soft. Did you make it? It looks handmade! It's been an eternity since we've had tea together." Walking slowly at *Comfort's* pace, we rattle off words in exhilaration. "So first, I'll put a kettle of water on, and then I'll show you to your room. I have the guest room back now that *Acceptance* has moved to the porch, oh, but you know that. Then we'll sit by the fire, enjoy some homemade muffins, and you can tell me what's happening in the world." Our sentences spill out like corn popping on an open flame. There's no doubt. Our reunion with *Comfort* is absolutely the best happening since our Loss.

With twinkling eyes, *Comfort* puts an arm around us as we begin strolling back up the path toward the house. She now slows her pace even more, which is to be expected when one is balancing a teapot on one's head, but we also sense that she is deep in thought. After a minute or so, *Comfort* stops to look at us. She studies our face with sympathetic eyes, and then, barely above a whisper, she says, "I know it has been so difficult, but I am here now."

She again puts her arm around our waist, and we continue our slow pace. We become overwhelmed with gratitude. Biting our lip, we battle at keeping ourselves from bursting into grateful tears. But there is no hiding our emotions from *Comfort.*

"Don't fight your tears, dear," she says gently.

And so we don't.

Once inside the house, we dry our eyes and become invigorated. "I'll heat the water and start baking the muffins," we tell her. "And oh, yes, I must pick flowers for your room—and then I will lay out my finest tea service! Later, I will think about dinner. I am so happy you are here!" we tell *Comfort* over and over again. "I just know you will never, *ever* leave!"

Oh, if only it were so.

Later in the evening, after tea, muffins, and a scrumptious dinner, we both sink deep into the couch by the fireplace to enjoy the warm glow of burning logs. A spring evening breeze floats through the open windows, causing a slight chill. In response, *Comfor*t unfolds the quilt and wraps it around us. We talk softly, reminiscing about the times we've had together, and how they abruptly ended with *Shock's* arrival. Our Loss seems so long ago now, and though the memories are still vivid, the stabbing pain is gone. We lean against *Comfort*'s shoulder with a deep sigh of relief. Drowsiness begins to overtake us, so we lay our head in her ample lap and she begins to stroke our hair. We hear soft music playing in the background and feel contentment. We have a wonderful sense for the first time since our Loss that—we are going to be okay.

The following morning, we wake up all *bright-eyed* and bushy-tailed. We are almost giddy as we prepare a breakfast of tea and biscuits. Renewed by our sense of well-being, we later pack a picnic basket in anticipation of a long, leisurely walk in the countryside with *Comfort* at our side.

By early afternoon, we find ourselves munching on nuts and fruit while lying contentedly on a blanket near a rushing stream. We marvel at the melodious sound of babbling water that has been absent from our world for so long. We notice the leaves budding profusely and wildflowers blooming. Brilliant hues of purple, yellow, and white crocus spread out across the distant meadow, reminiscent of *Comfort's* patchwork quilt. We see clouds billowing like white sails on a windy sea while the breeze murmurs in the branches above. There is no doubt that our mind is calmer, sharper, and less distracted.

A melody is tapping to the beat of our heart. Yes, life in all its wonder has returned. The passing of time has helped, but we would not be where we are except for the labor of our previous five friends who eventually brought us to *Comfort*.

Comfort seldom leaves us now, primarily, because we choose to keep her close. Each night, she wraps us up in peaceful dreams. The nightmares are gone. We dwell in pleasant memories, pushing away those that no longer help us—the haunting ones that lurk in dark corners. We sing long-forgotten songs. We notice the sentimental lyrics don't stab at our heart any longer. Not that long ago, we had to cover our ears when we would hear certain melodies. They were just too painful to hear. But that depth of despair has faded.

Gratefully, we bury the unhappy images of the past, along with the depression caused by the agonizing thoughts "if only" and "what could have been." We, with *Comfort's* companionship, choose to embrace the pleasures of now. We talk a lot. Sometimes, our words bring back the pain, but now, we can at least speak freely without our internal mirror shattering into pieces.

One afternoon, over tea, *Comfort* begins to talk about expanding our circle. She speaks of the need for others to be in our life and gently asks us if we would consider getting out more.

"But why?" we ask her. "I like our quiet time."

"There's more to life," she says. "And there are also more friends coming."

"More friends?" we ask, surprised. "There's more?" Then, without an ounce of hesitancy, we cry out, "Well, bring them on!"

Comfort promises she will.

More time passes by, and we start to become impatient as we anxiously anticipate the arrival of our new friends. Like children, we press our nose against the window watching the path.

"When are they coming? And will I recognize them?" we ask.

"They're coming soon. Yes, you'll recognize them," *Comfort* reassures us.

"Will they remember me?" we inquire.

Comfort throws up her hands. "Of course, they will remember you! Put your mind to rest! They have been waiting for some time now. They just want to make sure *you're* ready."

"So who are they?" we ask as we continue to stare out the window. *Comfort* has kept everything a secret.

"You will see," she says, smiling.

Admittedly, it feels like a century has passed by since we have given ourselves permission to enjoy life. But as we evaluate our state of being, we're confident we're ready. *Comfort*'s warm, healing presence has moved us forward, and we're now eager to be reacquainted with our next friends.

One afternoon as we are watching the path, we can't believe our eyes. Suddenly, we are ecstatic! We see them coming—at last! "They're here! They're here!" we yell.

One of them bursts through the door. The other crawls through the window. Music blares. Are those bagpipes? Oh my goodness! What an entrance!

"Hello, *Joy*! Hello *Laughter!*" we cry. "What took you guys so long?"

Joy and Laughter

Spring: Midday
White billowing clouds in blue sky
Flowers blooming, balloons,
and "Welcome Home" signs on house

What a scene! While continuing to play their bagpipes, *Joy* and *Laughter* march around our house triumphantly. We clap our hands in rhythm while marveling at their heavy knapsacks. Along with their bedrolls, they are overflowing with CDs, food, drinks, fishing rods, and various colors of Frisbees. We are filled with excitement as we anticipate the fun ahead of us—at long last!

Joy and *Laughter,* who are cousins, need no special pampering or even flowers in their room. In fact, they don't even need a room. Now that they are in, they take over the whole house. We are completely overwhelmed—but love every moment! As usual, we are fascinated by how they are dressed. Known to always be wearing some unexpected garb, we are not surprised to see them in plaid Scottish kilts, Ghillie shirts, woolen knee socks, and buckled shoes. There is no doubt: they have come to celebrate!

As they pound our back with excitement, the conversation between us is fast and furious, everyone's words tumbling into the others. "You look wonderful!" *Joy* exclaims. "Look at you—you are amazing! And I love that jacket you're wearing!" They patter on with their arms wrapped around our shoulders.

Laughter finds fluted glasses from his knapsack, then cracks open a bottle of bubbly. After filling the glasses, he raises his own and exclaims, "We missed you! Nothing has been the same while you were gone! We are so happy to be with you! Here's to friendship!" After we clink our glasses, sealing our reunion, *Joy* pulls out a CD from his knapsack and pops it into the stereo. "Come on," he yells, pushing the play button, "your favorite song! Let's dance!"

And so we do.

Wow! Never in a million years did we think that *Joy* and *Laughter* would ever find us again. But we were wrong. Every sentence, every phrase, rings a bell inside us. "Am I actually feeling happy?" we ask ourselves. "Can it be true? Are *Joy* and *Laughter* truly part of my life again? Can I have come back from being so far away? Can I trust these wonderful feelings? Are they for real?" We ponder for a few seconds—then shout out, "Yes, I can!"

Time doesn't just pass quickly; it whistles by like an arrow. The hours no longer drag; they practically trip over each other. There is simply not enough time in the day to do everything we want when we're hanging out with *Joy* and *Laughter*. We also notice that our moods are not as influenced by the whim of passing clouds. Early on, after our Loss, our burden would feel heavier on dark cloudy days. But now, *Joy* walks with us in the rain and *Laughte*r runs with us in the wind. Blue skies or gray, it doesn't matter. With *Joy* and *Laughter* at our side, life, once again, is good.

Before we know it, an entire season passes. Yet it seems like only yesterday when our two friends took over our house. We remember the first time their antics resulted in us rolling on the ground in laughter. We caught ourselves right in the middle of it. "Am I laughing?" we asked ourselves, "Is this a laugh? Did I just laugh out loud?" We were so grateful that we once again heard ourselves laugh; we shed tears of relief. It was incredible that we could feel—well, such pleasure!

Yes, it's true. Laughter is the best medicine. No other friends, not even our darling *Comfort* has made us feel this fulfilled, or this confident. And look at our face! Our color is back. The deep lines have disappeared. Our eyes are sparkling. Our smile is real, and we are happy for others, happy in the wonder of life, and happy in the knowledge that we made it through. Before long, we are riding bikes, going out to visit family and friends in their homes, shopping, and even offering to help others. We are playing games, going to movies, and enjoying long walks alone (without being lonely) because we know that when we get back home we will find *Comfort, Joy,* and *Laughter*. Yes, with these three friends, there is nothing more we need.

Oh, if only it were so.

With things going so smoothly, we can easily forget that happiness doesn't just flow on and on like Ol' Man River. This reality hits when one day we awaken to the fact that our honeymoon with *Joy* and *Laughte*r is fading. We still revel in the pleasure they brought us, but this pleasure no longer has the same intensity that it did in the beginning. We have been aware for a while now, that although we love *Joy* and *Laughter,* they can be a lot like oven-fresh chocolate-chip cookies, and we must be careful about over-indulging. Yes, when we are so filled up with *Joy* and *Laughter,* we often do not leave room for something of more, well, substance.

Before long, emptiness begins to creep in.

We've been dismissing for a while our need for something more, but lately, it's becoming more difficult to ignore. This uneasiness is difficult to describe but even harder to address. There is just a gnawing sense deep within us. Yes, there is no doubt, we've been denying it. However, we're now at a place where denial no longer works. "Doggone," we sigh.

Then one morning, we wake up and hear a familiar sound. Oh no! We immediately recognize the terrible squeaking sound of the porch swing. "How can that be?" we exclaim. We thought we were beyond that! "Calm down. Don't panic!" we tell ourselves. But try as we do, we cannot help feeling those old dreadful stabs of anxiety. We try once again to ignore them. A couple more days pass, and now we're sure—*Sob*, *Grief*, and *Sorrow* are peeking through the windows. They want back in.

Let's face it, the fabulous twosome, *Joy* and *Laughter*, have kept us from moving forward. We want them to be with us forever, and surely they will, but right now they are noisy and distracting, and we need to stop and listen. *Comfort* will know what to do. Of all of our friends, we trust her completely. We can always rely on her compassion and wise counsel. Yes, she will know what this nagging emptiness is all about.

And she does.

"*Comfort*," we ask one evening as we are together by the fire, our head in her lap. "I'm having anxiety about my Loss again. I thought it was behind me?"

Comfort nods. "I know," she says softly.

"Do you think I'm slipping backward? I thought I had done everything I was supposed to do. All eight friends have stayed in the house. I endured *Shock* and *Sob*. I tolerated *Grief* and *Sorrow*—and then I got used to them—but eventually pushed them out. I welcomed *Acceptance*, I battled with *Anger*, I adored you, and I squeezed everything I could out of *Joy* and *Laugher*. I feel like I am living again. So what's wrong? What am I missing?"

Comfort smiles and strokes our hair and says, "There is a ninth friend."

We are stunned. We instantly sit up and ask, "What? There is still another friend?"

"Yes, the last one," *Comfort* says calmly, aware of our alarm. She takes our hand. "Don't worry," *Comfort* reassures us. "She will be coming soon, now that you recognize something is missing. But you must realize that she is different than I am and also from the others. We all just showed up uninvited. This friend waits for an invitation."

"Will she come up the path?" we ask.

"No, dear, you'll have to go to her."

"But where is she?" we continue to probe.

"I can't tell you. You must find her on your own."

"But where do I look? How do I know she even exists?"

"Oh, she exists," *Comfort* assures us. "Throughout the ages, many great seers and renowned prophets have spoken about her, and for the most part, we are confident that all who seek her find her, although I'm afraid some might seek—but do not find."

Comfort ponders for a moment and then continues, her voice barely audible. "She dwells on a spiritual plane, and to find her, you must follow your heart. It will take some patience."

Not too many days after our conversation, we awake early. We pack up our bedroll, make some peanut butter and jelly sandwiches, grab a few apples, a thermos of tea, stuff it all into our knapsack, then walk out onto the porch and down the steps. It is here we pause and turn.

"What's her name?" we call back to *Comfort,* who's standing in the doorway.

"*Inner Peace*!" Comfort calls out.

We smile at *Sob, Grief, Sorrow,* and *Acceptance*, stretched out on the porch swing and rocking chairs. We nod as they wave at us. We then turn and walk down the path. We have made the decision. No matter how long it takes, we are going to find our ninth friend.

Inner Peace

Summer: Daylight
Bright sun, clear blue skies
Windows open, green grass, leaves, flowers at peak

How does one actually search for *Inner Peace*? Our other eight friends just showed up and took over. Why can't *Inner Peace* do the same? We walk to the end of the path and into the surrounding hills, all the while wrestling with the idea that *Inner Peace* dwells on a spiritual plane, and apparently, we find her by following our heart. However, we are consumed with questions.

"What if she's asleep?" we ask ourselves. "Are we supposed to awaken her? How do we do that? We can't just say, wake up! Or can we?" We have learned by now that none of our eight friends took orders very well. Another thought crosses our mind. Maybe *Inner Peace* is inside us and just can't get out.

"Okay!" we command. "Heart, brain, whichever, I want you to release *Inner Peace*!" We wait. Nothing happens. Apparently, it's not that simple—or is it?

That evening, we stop next to a tall pine tree, lay out our bedroll, and make a small fire. We sit and gaze at a spectacular sunset, and later, with birch logs crackling, we contemplate the myriad of stars gathered above like shining pinpricks in black velvet. The silvery scimitar of a moon hangs high in the west. We are awestruck by the grandeur of the night stage. How did all this magnificence come to be? We have an urge to applaud.

So we do.

During this time, we look around as we think we might find footsteps, but then, we remind ourselves that *Inner Peace* will not leave any tracks for us to follow. Nor as *Comfort* also confirmed, she isn't going to sneak up on us. After all, she is spiritual. We remember our last conversations with Comfort: "Can we hear her? Does she speak? Is she above us?" we probed. No, according to *Comfort*, we should be looking inward, not upward.

We continue to sit quietly, studying the stars, mesmerized by their secrets. We don't know how they came to be, but that's okay. We decide to just appreciate their wonder. Maybe it's the same with *Inner Peace*; we don't need to know all her charms or how she uses them. Maybe we're supposed to simply embrace her and accept her mysteries.

But first, we must find her.

The thought makes us anxious. What if we don't? *Comfort told* us that not everyone succeeds in their search for this ninth friend. So here we are, in the middle of the woods and we don't even know if we're heading in the right direction. We sigh deeply. "Will we ever find her?"

Months later, when we think back to that night, we still cannot articulate exactly what happened. We only know that we came out of the woods a different person than when we entered. We do not doubt the reality of the experience, but we are at a loss to describe what actually took place. Nonetheless, this is how we remember it:

We left our camp and began walking along a narrow path in the moonlight. We must have strayed from the trail, for we found ourselves in the midst of a heavy vapor circling the ground. We suddenly realized that we were standing at the edge of an abyss. We are visibly shaken as we cannot see the bottom nor can we see the other side. For one fearful moment, we are rooted in place. We call out for help. Immediately, a sense of calmness comes over us. The calmness is accompanied by a heightened sense of security—suddenly, the fear is gone. Courage emerges and an inner voice tells us that we must cross over. We trust the voice and then—we leap! Not physically, mind you, but with our mind and our heart.

And now—here we are, on the other side.

A feeling of solitude, deeper than we've ever known, comes over us. We are in a space so quiet, so calm, that all we hear is our breathing. Wait, not just our breathing—we hear something else, a faraway voice, but it's too faint to make out. We move toward it, but the voice moves as well, like a moth flitting back and forth in the night—now nearby, now farther away. We concentrate on it, completely entranced. Intrigue, confusion, and excitement all stumble over each other as they roll around in our mind. Yet our overwhelming feeling is one of harmony.

The voice becomes melodic, but still no louder than a whisper. It's very close. Now it's next to us. We slowly turn toward the voice, careful not to frighten it off. Yearning to connect, we reach out to touch it. Instantly, the voice changes into a beautiful, feminine seraph. At first, we don't move. We are captivated by the radiance of her dark skin and long, white, curly hair. We step closer. Then we see that in the palm of her hand, she holds a golden flickering flame that illuminates the surrounding night with a soft glow. The image takes our breath away. The world pauses, for just a second, waiting for us to catch up. We're trembling, and our voice is barely audible.

"Hi, *Inner Peace!*"

With a beautiful smile as warm as a summer breeze, *Inner Peace* gently takes our hand and the dancing flame jumps from her palm to ours, creating a calm, warming sensation. Her melodious voice whispers, "Forgive yourself."

Guilt that has burdened our spirit since our Loss falls away like a broken chain. For so long, we had been prisoners of our regrets. Letting go of this torment breaks its control over us. The twirling flame now burns brighter.

Inner Peace's soft voice whispers again, "Do not judge others."

We are seized by an intense desire to make amends to those who we've hurt. We call out their names, one by one, asking for forgiveness. We release them, along with the pain we have held for so long. Another link breaks, and more chains clink to the ground. We are overwhelmed by feelings of serenity. Taking a deep breath, not lifting our eyes from the soothing flame, we move as close as we can to *Inner Peace*. We feel *her* breath upon us.

"Do not allow bitterness into your world." *Her* voice grows stronger. "Release it. The path to peace is compassion."

Freedom! For the first time since our Loss, the gut-wrenching question, "Why me—why did this happen to me?" is no longer relevant; it disappears along with everything else that's beyond our control. *Clink*. The remaining chains fall away.

The flame continues to dance in our hand, and *Inner Peace's* voice now becomes so strong it leaves an echo. "Love yourself. Love all who you know." Our obsessions with the past, our fears and anxiety for the future, vanish—as does the flame.

The luminance of *Inner Peace* spreads throughout our entire being. We reach out to *her* and *she* embraces us. Suddenly, we're in a narrow river, floating in a slow-moving current. We close our eyes and let the current take us where it will. We don't try to grab an overhead branch or swim to shore. We float in peace.

That is how we remember it.

As more seasons pass, calm has replaced anxiety. Love for ourselves and others now grace our life, providing an ideal environment for *Acceptance, Comfort, Joy,* and *Laughter. Sob* only enters now and then. She, too, will always be with us. And now, we welcome her when she knocks.

We still stumble over what to say when people comment, "You look different. Something has come over you. What is it?" We are at a loss to explain this mystical reconciliation between our mind, body, and soul. We doubt that will ever change. We tell ourselves that perhaps it's an awakening, enlightenment, or maybe a new realization that we are not alone. Or it might be the absence of guilt or having made amends with others. Whatever it is, our fear is gone. We remain actively engaged with the world, but our physical self—our emotions, our worries—no longer consume us. Our mind still spins at times with what-ifs, but they no longer escalate. We have settled in.

Reconciling our Loss through *Inner Peace* is an incredible experience, so astounding that we come to believe that *Inner Peace* is a spiritual gift, just like *Comfort* said. We are immensely grateful, knowing this gift would never be ours without our other eight friends— eight devoted friends—who, all along, were partners in the larger plan designed to lead us to the ninth.

Over time, we continue to integrate *Inner Peace* into our total being. Yes, we are convinced we will never again feel anxiety, fear, or anger. We will never again let Loss take over our life. We will never again struggle with keeping our *Inner Peace*.

Oh, if only it were so.

Epilogue

If you never before believed in the existence of a master plan or its Architect, after reading about our magnificent nine friends, perhaps you might consider it. But regardless whether you believe or not, the next time Loss strikes, remember that you are not meant to walk its long difficult path alone. You can always count on having a friend or two or three—to walk with you. Managing Loss is life's greatest challenge. How proficient we become very often determines our overall feelings of well-being. So tuck this little book away. You will need it again.

To those of you who opened the door to the ninth friend, *Inner Peace*, you have a lifelong advantage. The next time you experience Loss, *Inner Peace* provides you with the assurance that you will survive. There is also consolation in knowing that with this ninth friend, your journey to healing is shorter.

Unfortunately, no one possesses *Inner Peace* every moment of their life. There is just too much hardship and pain in our world not to notice. And for those with empathy and compassion, maintaining a constant state of serenity is impossible. However, even if *Inner Peace* at times appears distant, she is never far away—and that is the good news.

The other good news is that no one can *ever* take her from you. Indeed, *Inner Peace* is the only Loss you will never experience. She is with you forever and ever. Amen. Ameen. Om. Selah.

It is so.